PARKINSON'S DISEASE COOKBOOK

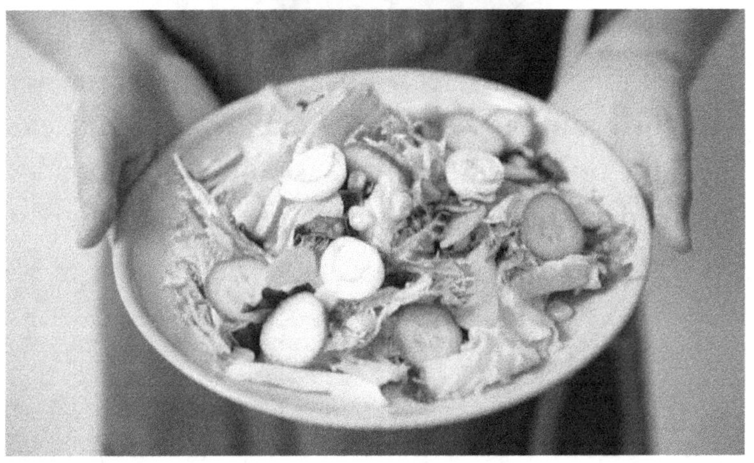

A Practical Guide to Crafting Delicious, Nutrient-Dense Meals for Parkinson's Disease Management

BY

MICHELLE T. RILLS

About the book

The "Parkinson's Disease Cookbook" is a comprehensive guide designed to support individuals living with Parkinson's disease in maintaining a healthy and balanced diet. Written with the specific dietary needs and challenges of Parkinson's patients in mind, this book offers a wealth of practical information, delicious recipes, and valuable tips to help manage symptoms and improve overall well-being.

At its core, the cookbook provides an introduction to Parkinson's disease and its relationship to nutrition, helping readers understand how dietary choices can impact symptoms and quality of life. It offers insights into the nutrients that are particularly beneficial for individuals with Parkinson's, as well as those that should be consumed in moderation.

The book is divided into sections that cover every aspect of meal planning and preparation, from breakfast to dinner, snacks, and beverages. Each section includes a variety of recipes carefully crafted to meet the nutritional needs of Parkinson's patients while also being delicious and easy to prepare.

Whether it's a hearty breakfast to start the day, a nutritious lunch to sustain energy levels, or a comforting dinner to unwind in the evening, the cookbook offers options to suit every taste and dietary preference.

In addition to recipes, the cookbook also provides practical advice on grocery shopping, kitchen organization, and meal modification for those with specific dietary restrictions or preferences. It emphasizes the importance of a well-rounded diet and offers guidance on incorporating healthy habits into everyday life to support overall health and symptom management.

With its wealth of accessible information and mouthwatering recipes, the "Parkinson's Disease Cookbook" is an invaluable resource for individuals with Parkinson's, their caregivers, and anyone looking to support their loved ones on their journey to better health through nutrition.

Table of Contents

Introduction to Parkinson's Disease and Nutrition

The "Introduction to Parkinson's Disease and Nutrition" serves as the foundational chapter in the Parkinson's Disease Cookbook, providing readers with essential information about the relationship between Parkinson's disease and dietary choices.

This section begins by offering a comprehensive overview of Parkinson's disease, including its symptoms, progression, and impact on daily life. It explains the underlying causes of Parkinson's, such as the loss of dopamine-producing cells in the brain, and how these changes can affect various aspects of health, including motor function, cognition, and mood.

The chapter then delves into the role of nutrition in managing Parkinson's symptoms and supporting overall well-being. It highlights the importance of a balanced diet rich in essential nutrients, vitamins, and minerals for maintaining optimal health, particularly in individuals with Parkinson's.

Readers are introduced to specific dietary considerations for Parkinson's patients, such as the potential impact of certain medications on appetite and digestion, as well as common nutritional deficiencies associated with the disease. Emphasis is placed on the importance of maintaining a healthy weight, managing constipation, and staying hydrated, all of which can have a significant impact on symptom management and quality of life.

Furthermore, the chapter discusses the potential benefits of specific nutrients and dietary components for individuals with Parkinson's, such as antioxidants, omega-3 fatty acids, and protein, in mitigating symptoms and slowing disease progression.

Overall, the "Introduction to Parkinson's Disease and Nutrition" sets the stage for the rest of the cookbook by providing readers with a solid understanding of the importance of nutrition in managing Parkinson's disease. It empowers individuals with knowledge and resources to make informed dietary choices that can positively impact their health and well-being.

Chapter 2

Understanding Dietary Needs for Parkinson's Patients

Understanding Dietary Needs for Parkinson's Patients" is a critical section in the Parkinson's Disease Cookbook, aimed at elucidating the specific nutritional requirements and challenges faced by individuals living with Parkinson's disease.

This segment starts by delineating the unique dietary considerations that arise due to Parkinson's disease, such as changes in metabolism, medication interactions, and motor impairments affecting eating and swallowing. It emphasizes the importance of a tailored diet that addresses these challenges while promoting overall health and well-being.

Key dietary needs for Parkinson's patients are explored in detail, including:

1. Maintaining Adequate Nutrition: Due to potential difficulties with appetite, chewing, and swallowing, ensuring sufficient caloric intake and nutrient absorption is paramount.

2. Balancing Macronutrients: Proper distribution of carbohydrates, proteins, and fats is essential for energy levels, muscle function, and overall health. The section discusses recommended proportions and sources of each macronutrient.

3. Micronutrient Supplementation: Parkinson's disease can lead to deficiencies in certain vitamins and minerals, such as vitamin D, B vitamins, and antioxidants. Strategies for supplementing these nutrients through diet and/or supplements are addressed.

4. Hydration: Parkinson's patients may experience dehydration due to reduced thirst sensation or medication side effects. Tips for maintaining adequate hydration levels are provided.

5. Fiber and Digestive Health: Constipation is a common issue in Parkinson's disease, necessitating a diet rich in fiber and hydration to promote regular bowel movements.

6. Medication Management: Some foods and beverages can interact with Parkinson's medications, affecting absorption and efficacy. Guidance on timing meals and medications is offered to optimize treatment outcomes.

Overall, "Understanding Dietary Needs for Parkinson's Patients" equips readers with the knowledge and tools to address nutritional challenges associated with Parkinson's disease. By tailoring their diet to meet specific needs, individuals can better manage symptoms, improve overall health, and enhance their quality of life.

Chapter 3

Tips for Meal Planning and Preparation

Tips for Meal Planning and Preparation is a pivotal section within the Parkinson's Disease Cookbook, offering practical guidance to streamline the process of creating nutritious and enjoyable meals while accommodating the unique needs and challenges associated with Parkinson's disease.

1. Set Realistic Goals: Begin by establishing realistic meal planning goals based on individual preferences, dietary restrictions, and energy levels. Break down large tasks into manageable steps to alleviate stress and overwhelm.

2. Create a Weekly Meal Schedule: Plan meals for the week ahead, taking into account factors such as dietary requirements, convenience, and variety. Incorporate a balance of protein, carbohydrates, and healthy fats into each meal to support overall health and energy levels.

3. Prep Ingredients in Advance: To minimize cooking time and effort, pre-chop vegetables, marinate proteins, and portion out ingredients in advance. Utilize time-saving kitchen tools and techniques, such as slow cookers, batch cooking, and one-pot meals.

4. Opt for Simple and Nutrient-Dense Recipes: Choose recipes that are easy to prepare and require minimal cooking skills, such as soups, stews, and stir-fries. Focus on incorporating nutrient-dense ingredients, such as whole grains, lean proteins, and colorful fruits and vegetables, to maximize nutritional benefits.

5. Consider Texture Modifications: For individuals with swallowing difficulties or impaired motor skills, consider modifying food textures to make meals easier to chew and swallow. Experiment with pureed, minced, or soft foods, and use sauces or gravies to add moisture and flavor.

6. Mealtime Environment: Create a comfortable and conducive mealtime environment by minimizing distractions, such as television or electronic devices, and focusing on enjoying the sensory experience of eating. Encourage relaxed and unhurried eating to aid digestion and promote satisfaction.

7. Stay Hydrated: Remember to include hydrating beverages, such as water, herbal teas, or infused water, alongside meals to maintain optimal hydration levels throughout the day.

8. Adapt and Modify as Needed: Be flexible and willing to adapt meal plans and recipes based on individual preferences, appetite fluctuations, and symptom management. Listen to your body's cues and make adjustments as needed to ensure a balanced and enjoyable eating experience.

By implementing these practical tips for meal planning and preparation, individuals with Parkinson's disease can simplify the cooking process, optimize nutrition, and enhance their overall well-being.

Chapter 4

Breakfast Recipes for Balanced Nutrition and Energy

1. Avocado Toast with Poached Egg:

Ingredients: Whole grain bread, avocado, eggs, salt, pepper, lemon juice.

Method: Toast bread, mash avocado with lemon juice, spread on toast, poach egg, place on top of avocado, season with salt and pepper.

2. Spinach and Mushroom Omelette:

Ingredients: Eggs, spinach, mushrooms, onion, garlic, olive oil, salt, pepper.

Method: Sauté onions and garlic in olive oil, add mushrooms and spinach, cook until wilted, pour beaten eggs over vegetables, cook until set, fold and serve.

3. Greek Yogurt Parfait with Berries and Almonds:

Ingredients: Greek yogurt, mixed berries, almonds, honey.

Method: Layer yogurt, berries, and almonds in a glass, drizzle with honey.

4. Banana Walnut Pancakes:

Ingredients: Whole wheat flour, banana, walnuts, eggs, milk, baking powder, cinnamon, salt.

Method: Mash banana, mix with eggs and milk, add dry ingredients, fold in chopped walnuts, cook pancakes on a griddle until golden.

5. Quinoa Breakfast Bowl with Fruit and Nuts:

Ingredients: Cooked quinoa, mixed fruit (such as berries, banana, and apple), almonds, honey.

Method: Mix quinoa with fruit and almonds, drizzle with honey.

6. Oatmeal with Chia Seeds and Blueberries:
Ingredients: Rolled oats, chia seeds, blueberries, almond milk, honey.

Method: Cook oats with almond milk, stir in chia seeds, top with blueberries and honey.

7. Whole Grain Breakfast Burrito:
Ingredients: Whole grain tortilla, scrambled eggs, black beans, salsa, avocado, spinach.

Method: Fill tortilla with scrambled eggs, black beans, salsa, avocado, and spinach, roll up and serve.

8. Sweet Potato Hash with Turkey Sausage:
Ingredients: Sweet potatoes, turkey sausage, onion, bell pepper, olive oil, salt, pepper, paprika.

Method: Sauté onions and bell pepper in olive oil, add diced sweet potatoes and turkey sausage, cook until tender, season with salt, pepper, and paprika.

9. Fruit Smoothie with Spinach and Flaxseeds:

Ingredients: Spinach, mixed fruit (such as berries and banana), flaxseeds, Greek yogurt, almond milk.

Method: Blend spinach, fruit, flaxseeds, yogurt, and almond milk until smooth.

10. Egg and Veggie Muffin Cups:

Ingredients: Eggs, bell peppers, onion, spinach, cherry tomatoes, feta cheese, salt, pepper.

Method: Whisk eggs with salt and pepper, mix in chopped vegetables and feta cheese, pour into muffin cups, bake until set.

11. Smoked Salmon and Cream Cheese Bagel:

Ingredients: Whole grain bagel, smoked salmon, cream cheese, cucumber slices, dill.

Method: Toast bagel, spread cream cheese, top with smoked salmon, cucumber slices, and dill.

12. Egg and Spinach Breakfast Wrap:

Ingredients: Whole grain wrap, eggs, spinach, cherry tomatoes, feta cheese, olive oil, salt, pepper.

Method: Scramble eggs with spinach, tomatoes, and feta cheese, place in a wrap, fold and serve.

13. Coconut Chia Seed Pudding with Mango:

Ingredients: Chia seeds, coconut milk, mango, honey.

Method: Mix chia seeds with coconut milk and honey, refrigerate until set, top with diced mango.

14. Whole Grain Waffles with Fresh Fruit:

Ingredients: Whole grain waffle mix, mixed fruit (such as berries and banana), maple syrup.

Method: Prepare waffles according to package instructions, top with fresh fruit and maple syrup.

15. Almond Butter and Banana Smoothie:

Ingredients: Almond butter, banana, almond milk, Greek yogurt, honey.

Method: Blend almond butter, banana, almond milk, yogurt, and honey until smooth.

16. Turmeric Scrambled Tofu:

Ingredients: Firm tofu, turmeric, onion, bell pepper, spinach, olive oil, salt, pepper.

Method: Crumble tofu, sauté with onions, peppers, and spinach in olive oil, season with turmeric, salt, and pepper.

17. Berry Quinoa Breakfast Bowl:

Ingredients: Cooked quinoa, mixed berries, almond slices, honey.

Method: Mix quinoa with berries and almonds, drizzle with honey.

18. Apple Cinnamon Overnight Oats:

Ingredients: Rolled oats, apple, cinnamon, almond milk, maple syrup.

Method: Mix oats, diced apple, cinnamon, almond milk, and maple syrup in a jar, refrigerate overnight, serve cold.

19. Turkey and Veggie Breakfast Skillet:

Ingredients: Ground turkey, bell peppers, onion, spinach, garlic, eggs, olive oil, salt, pepper.

Method:
Sauté turkey with onions, peppers, and garlic in olive oil, add spinach and crack eggs over the top, cook until eggs are set.

20. Green Tea Smoothie with Spinach and Pineapple:

Ingredients: Spinach, pineapple, banana, green tea, Greek yogurt, honey.

Method: Blend spinach, pineapple, banana, green tea, yogurt, and honey until smooth.

Chapter 5

Lunch Ideas for Sustained Energy Throughout the Day

1. Quinoa Salad with Chickpeas and Avocado:

Ingredients: Cooked quinoa, chickpeas, diced avocado, cherry tomatoes, cucumber, red onion, lemon juice, olive oil, salt, pepper.

Method: Combine all ingredients in a bowl, toss gently, and serve.

2. Mediterranean Veggie Wrap:

Ingredients: Whole grain wrap, hummus, mixed greens, sliced cucumber, bell peppers, cherry tomatoes, feta cheese, olives.

Method: Spread hummus on the wrap, add veggies and feta cheese, wrap tightly, and enjoy.

3. Grilled Chicken and Vegetable Skewers:

Ingredients: Chicken breast, bell peppers, zucchini, red onion, olive oil, lemon juice, garlic, oregano, salt, pepper.

Method: Marinate chicken and vegetables, skewer them, grill until cooked through, and serve with a side salad.

4. Salmon and Quinoa Bowl:

Ingredients: Grilled salmon, cooked quinoa, steamed broccoli, sliced avocado, shredded carrots, sesame seeds, soy sauce.

Method: Arrange ingredients in a bowl, drizzle with soy sauce, and sprinkle sesame seeds on top.

5. Turkey and Veggie Lettuce Wraps:

Ingredients: Romaine lettuce leaves, sliced turkey breast, sliced cucumber, shredded carrots, avocado, hummus.

Method: Fill lettuce leaves with turkey, veggies, and hummus, roll up, and enjoy.

6. Greek Salad with Grilled Chicken:

Ingredients: Grilled chicken breast, romaine lettuce, cherry tomatoes, cucumber, red onion, kalamata olives, feta cheese, Greek dressing.

Method: Toss all ingredients with Greek dressing and serve.

7. Vegetarian Quinoa Stuffed Bell Peppers:

Ingredients: Bell peppers, cooked quinoa, black beans, corn, diced tomatoes, shredded cheese, taco seasoning.

Method: Stuff bell peppers with quinoa mixture, top with cheese, bake until peppers are tender, and serve.

8. Asian-Inspired Tofu Stir-Fry:

Ingredients: Firm tofu, mixed vegetables (such as broccoli, bell peppers, snap peas), soy sauce, garlic, ginger, sesame oil, rice vinegar.

Method: Sauté tofu and vegetables in sesame oil, add garlic and ginger, stir in soy sauce and rice vinegar, and serve over brown rice.

9. Caprese Salad with Whole Grain Bread:
Ingredients: Fresh mozzarella cheese, sliced tomatoes, fresh basil leaves, whole grain bread, balsamic glaze.

Method: Layer mozzarella, tomato, and basil on whole grain bread, drizzle with balsamic glaze, and enjoy.

10. Tuna Salad Lettuce Wraps:
Ingredients: Canned tuna, Greek yogurt, diced celery, diced red onion, lemon juice, Dijon mustard, lettuce leaves.

Method: Mix tuna salad ingredients, spoon onto lettuce leaves, roll up, and serve.

11. Sweet Potato and Black Bean Quesadillas:
Ingredients: Whole grain tortillas, mashed sweet potatoes, black beans, diced bell peppers, shredded cheese, cumin, chili powder.

Method: Spread sweet potatoes on tortillas, top with black beans, bell peppers, cheese, and spices, fold in half, and cook until crispy.

12. Shrimp and Veggie Stir-Fry:

Ingredients: Shrimp, mixed vegetables (such as bell peppers, broccoli, carrots), garlic, ginger, soy sauce, sesame oil, brown rice.

Method: Sauté shrimp and vegetables in sesame oil with garlic and ginger, stir in soy sauce, and serve over brown rice.

13. Chicken Caesar Salad Wrap:

Ingredients: Grilled chicken breast, romaine lettuce, Caesar dressing, shredded Parmesan cheese, whole grain wrap.

Method: Fill wrap with chicken, lettuce, Caesar dressing, and Parmesan cheese, roll up, and enjoy.

14. Mango Chicken Salad:

Ingredients: Grilled chicken breast, mixed greens, diced mango, sliced avocado, sliced almonds, balsamic vinaigrette.

Method: Toss all ingredients with balsamic vinaigrette and serve.

15. Vegetable and Lentil Soup:

Ingredients: Lentils, mixed vegetables (such as carrots, celery, onions), garlic, vegetable broth, diced tomatoes, Italian seasoning.

Method: Cook lentils and vegetables in broth with tomatoes and seasoning until tender, and serve hot.

16. Chicken and Vegetable Quinoa Bowl:

Ingredients: Cooked quinoa, grilled chicken breast, steamed broccoli, roasted sweet potatoes, cherry tomatoes, avocado, tahini dressing (tahini, lemon juice, garlic, water), salt, pepper.

Method: Arrange cooked quinoa, grilled chicken breast, steamed broccoli, roasted sweet potatoes, halved cherry tomatoes, and sliced avocado in a bowl. Drizzle with tahini dressing. Season with salt and pepper to taste.

17. Turkey and Spinach Salad with Cranberry Vinaigrette:

Ingredients: Sliced turkey breast, baby spinach, dried cranberries, sliced almonds, feta cheese, cranberry vinaigrette (cranberry juice, olive oil, apple cider vinegar, Dijon mustard, honey), salt, pepper.

Method: Arrange baby spinach on a plate. Top with sliced turkey breast, dried cranberries, sliced almonds, and crumbled feta cheese. Drizzle with cranberry vinaigrette. Season with salt and pepper to taste.

18. Mediterranean Chickpea Wrap:

Ingredients: Whole grain wrap, hummus, cooked chickpeas, cucumber slices, cherry tomatoes, Kalamata olives, feta cheese, fresh parsley, lemon juice, olive oil, salt, pepper.

Method: Spread hummus on a whole grain wrap. Layer cooked chickpeas, cucumber slices, halved cherry tomatoes, sliced Kalamata olives, crumbled feta cheese, and chopped fresh parsley on top. Drizzle with lemon juice and olive oil. Season with salt and pepper. Roll up and serve.

19. Asian Tofu Salad with Peanut Dressing:

Ingredients: Firm tofu, mixed greens, shredded carrots, sliced cucumber, edamame, red bell pepper, green onions, cilantro, peanuts, peanut dressing (peanut butter, soy sauce, rice vinegar, honey, ginger, garlic, sesame oil).

Method: Press tofu to remove excess , then dice into cubes. Sauté tofu until golden brown. Arrange mixed greens on a plate. Top with shredded carrots, sliced cucumber, edamame, sliced red bell pepper, diced green onions, chopped cilantro, and sautéed tofu. Drizzle with peanut dressing. Garnish with chopped peanuts.

20. Shrimp and Avocado Salad:

Ingredients: Cooked shrimp, avocado, mixed greens, cherry tomatoes, cucumber, red onion, lemon vinaigrette (lemon juice, olive oil, Dijon mustard, honey), salt, pepper.

Method: Arrange mixed greens on a plate. Top with cooked shrimp, sliced avocado, halved cherry tomatoes, sliced cucumber, and thinly sliced red onion. Drizzle with lemon vinaigrette. Season with salt and pepper to taste.

Chapter 6

Dinner Recipes to Support Overall Health and Well-being

1. Grilled Lemon Herb Chicken:
Ingredients: Chicken breasts, lemon juice, olive oil, garlic, fresh herbs (such as thyme, rosemary, parsley), salt, pepper.

Method: Marinate chicken breasts in a mixture of lemon juice, olive oil, minced garlic, chopped herbs, salt, and pepper. Grill until cooked through and serve with steamed vegetables and quinoa.

2. Baked Salmon with Roasted Vegetables:
Ingredients: Salmon filets, olive oil, lemon juice, garlic powder, paprika, mixed vegetables (such as broccoli, bell peppers, carrots), salt, pepper.

Method: Season salmon filets with olive oil, lemon juice, garlic powder, paprika, salt, and pepper. Bake in the oven until cooked through. Serve with roasted mixed vegetables.

3. Vegetable Stir-Fry with Tofu:

Ingredients: Firm tofu, mixed vegetables (such as bell peppers, broccoli, snap peas, carrots), garlic, ginger, soy sauce, sesame oil, cooked brown rice.

Method: Sauté tofu until golden brown. Add minced garlic and ginger, followed by mixed vegetables. Cook until vegetables are tender-crisp. Add soy sauce and sesame oil. Serve over cooked brown rice.

4. Turkey and Quinoa Stuffed Bell Peppers:

Ingredients: Bell peppers, ground turkey, cooked quinoa, diced tomatoes, onion, garlic, chili powder, cumin, shredded cheese, cilantro.

Method: Cook ground turkey with diced onions, minced garlic, chili powder, and cumin. Mix cooked quinoa, diced tomatoes, cooked turkey mixture, and shredded cheese. Stuff bell peppers with the mixture. Bake until peppers are tender and cheese is melted. Garnish with chopped cilantro.

5. Vegetarian Lentil Soup:

Ingredients: Lentils, vegetable broth, diced tomatoes, carrots, celery, onion, garlic, bay leaves, thyme, spinach, lemon juice, salt, pepper.

Method: Sauté diced onions, carrots, and celery until softened. Add minced garlic, lentils, diced tomatoes, bay leaves, thyme, and vegetable broth. Simmer until lentils are tender. Stir in spinach and lemon juice. Season with salt and pepper.

6. Shrimp and Broccoli Stir-Fry:

Ingredients: Shrimp, broccoli florets, bell peppers, onion, garlic, ginger, soy sauce, honey, sesame oil, cooked brown rice.

Method: Sauté shrimp until pink and cooked through. Add minced garlic and ginger, followed by broccoli florets, sliced bell peppers, and diced onions. Stir in soy sauce, honey, and sesame oil. Serve over cooked brown rice.

7. Mediterranean Chickpea Salad:

Ingredients: Chickpeas, cucumber, cherry tomatoes, red onion, Kalamata olives, feta cheese, olive oil, lemon juice, dried oregano, salt, pepper.

Method: Combine chickpeas, chopped cucumber, halved cherry tomatoes, thinly sliced red onion, Kalamata olives, and crumbled feta cheese. Dress with olive oil, lemon juice, dried oregano, salt, and pepper.

8. Teriyaki Tofu Stir-Fry:

Ingredients: Firm tofu, mixed vegetables (such as bell peppers, broccoli, carrots), garlic, ginger, teriyaki sauce, cooked quinoa or brown rice.

Method: Sauté tofu until golden brown. Add minced garlic and ginger, followed by mixed vegetables. Cook until vegetables are tender-crisp. Stir in teriyaki sauce. Serve over cooked quinoa or brown rice.

9. Lemon Garlic Herb Roasted Chicken:

Ingredients: Chicken thighs or breasts, lemon zest, garlic, fresh herbs (such as rosemary, thyme, parsley), olive oil, salt, pepper.

Method: Mix lemon zest, minced garlic, chopped herbs, olive oil, salt, and pepper. Rub the mixture over chicken thighs or breasts. Roast until cooked through and serve with roasted vegetables.

10. Vegetable and Bean Chili:

Ingredients: Mixed beans (such as kidney beans, black beans, pinto beans), diced tomatoes, bell peppers, onion, garlic, chili powder, cumin, paprika, vegetable broth, corn, cilantro, lime wedges, avocado.

Method: Sauté diced onions, bell peppers, and minced garlic until softened. Add mixed beans, diced tomatoes, chili powder, cumin, paprika, and vegetable broth. Simmer until flavors meld. Stir in corn and chopped cilantro. Serve with lime wedges and sliced avocado.

11. Miso Glazed Salmon with Stir-Fried Vegetables:

Ingredients: Salmon filets, miso paste, soy sauce, maple syrup, garlic, ginger, mixed vegetables (such as bell peppers, broccoli, snap peas, carrots), sesame oil, cooked brown rice.

Method: Mix miso paste, soy sauce, maple syrup, minced garlic, and grated ginger. Brush over salmon filets and bake until cooked through. Stir-fry mixed vegetables in sesame oil until tender-crisp. Serve salmon with stir-fried vegetables and cooked brown rice.

12. Caprese Stuffed Chicken Breast:

Ingredients: Chicken breasts, mozzarella cheese, cherry tomatoes, fresh basil leaves, balsamic glaze, olive oil, salt, pepper.

Method: Cut a pocket into each chicken breast. Stuff with sliced mozzarella cheese, halved cherry tomatoes, and fresh basil leaves. Season with salt and pepper. Drizzle with olive oil. Bake until chicken is cooked through. Serve with a drizzle of balsamic glaze.

13. Turkey and Vegetable Stir-Fry:

Ingredients: Ground turkey, mixed vegetables (such as bell peppers, broccoli, carrots), garlic, ginger, soy sauce, hoisin sauce, sesame oil, cooked quinoa or brown rice.

Method: Sauté ground turkey until cooked through. Add minced garlic and ginger, followed by mixed vegetables. Cook until vegetables are tender-crisp. Stir in soy sauce, hoisin sauce, and sesame oil. Serve over cooked quinoa or brown rice.

14. Vegetarian Stuffed Zucchini Boats:

Ingredients: Zucchini, cooked quinoa, black beans, corn, diced tomatoes, onion, garlic, chili powder, cumin, shredded cheese, cilantro.

Method: Cut zucchini in half lengthwise and scoop out the seeds to create boats. Mix cooked quinoa, black beans, corn, diced tomatoes, diced onions, minced garlic, chili powder, cumin, and shredded cheese. Stuffed zucchini boats with the mixture. Bake until zucchini is tender and cheese is melted. Garnish with chopped cilantro.

15. Honey Garlic Shrimp with Broccoli:

Ingredients: Shrimp, broccoli florets, garlic, honey, soy sauce, ginger, sesame oil, cooked brown rice.

Method: Sauté shrimp until pink and cooked through. Remove from the pan. Sauté broccoli florets in minced garlic until tender-crisp. Return shrimp to the pan. Stir in honey, soy sauce, grated ginger, and sesame oil. Serve over cooked brown rice.

16. Lemon Herb Roasted Vegetables:

Ingredients: Assorted vegetables (such as carrots, potatoes, Brussels sprouts, cauliflower), olive oil, lemon juice, garlic, fresh herbs (such as thyme, rosemary), salt, pepper.

Method: Toss assorted vegetables with olive oil, lemon juice, minced garlic, chopped herbs, salt, and pepper. Roast until tender and golden brown.

17. Black Bean and Sweet Potato Enchiladas:

Ingredients: Black beans, sweet potatoes, bell peppers, onion, garlic, cumin, chili powder, corn tortillas, enchilada sauce, shredded cheese, avocado, cilantro.

Method: Sauté diced sweet potatoes, bell peppers, onions, and minced garlic until tender. Add black beans, cumin, and chili powder. Fill corn tortillas with the sweet potato mixture. Roll up and place in a baking dish. Pour enchilada sauce over the top and sprinkle with shredded cheese. Bake until bubbly and cheese is melted. Serve with sliced avocado and chopped cilantro.

18. Salmon and Asparagus Foil Packets:

Ingredients: Salmon filets, asparagus spears, lemon slices, garlic, fresh dill, olive oil, salt, pepper.

Method: Place salmon filets and asparagus spears on a piece of foil. Top with lemon slices, minced garlic, chopped fresh dill, olive oil, salt, and pepper. Seal the foil packets and bake until salmon is cooked through and asparagus is tender.

19. Vegetable and Tofu Pad Thai:

Ingredients: Rice noodles, tofu, mixed vegetables (such as bell peppers, carrots, bean sprouts), garlic, ginger, soy sauce, tamarind paste, lime juice, peanuts, green onions, cilantro.

Method: Cook rice noodles according to package instructions. Sauté cubed tofu until golden brown. Add minced garlic and ginger, followed by mixed vegetables. Stir in cooked rice noodles, soy sauce, tamarind paste, and lime juice. Serve garnished with chopped peanuts, sliced green onions, and chopped cilantro.

20. Eggplant Parmesan:

Ingredients: Eggplant, breadcrumbs, grated Parmesan cheese, eggs, marinara sauce, mozzarella cheese, fresh basil, olive oil, salt, pepper.

Method: Slice eggplant into rounds and dip in beaten eggs, then coat in a mixture of breadcrumbs and grated Parmesan cheese. Fry until golden brown. Layer fried eggplant slices with marinara sauce, shredded mozzarella cheese, and fresh basil leaves. Bake until the cheese is melted and bubbly.

These dinner recipes offer a variety of flavors and nutrients to support overall health and well-being. Enjoy experimenting with these wholesome and delicious meals!

Chapter 7

Snack Options for Quick and Healthy Boosts

1. Mixed Nuts: A handful of mixed nuts like almonds, walnuts, and cashews provide healthy fats, protein, and fiber for a satisfying snack.

2. Greek Yogurt with Berries: Greek yogurt topped with fresh berries is rich in protein, calcium, and antioxidants.

3. Apple Slices with Peanut Butter: Apple slices paired with peanut butter offer a balance of carbohydrates, healthy fats, and protein.

4. Carrot Sticks with Hummus: Carrot sticks dipped in hummus provide a crunchy, satisfying snack packed with fiber and protein.

5. Hard-Boiled Eggs: Hard-boiled eggs are convenient and rich in protein, vitamins, and minerals.

6. Edamame: Steamed edamame pods are a nutritious snack high in protein, fiber, and essential nutrients.

7. Cottage Cheese with Pineapple: Cottage cheese paired with pineapple chunks offers a blend of protein and vitamin C.

8. Whole Grain Crackers with Avocado: Whole grain crackers topped with mashed avocado are a source of healthy fats, fiber, and vitamins.

9. Trail Mix: A mix of nuts, seeds, and dried fruits provides energy-boosting nutrients and satisfies hunger on-the-go.

10. Sliced Cucumber with Hummus: Cucumber slices dipped in hummus offer a hydrating and nutritious snack option.

11. Yogurt Parfait: Layer Greek yogurt with granola and sliced fruits like strawberries or bananas for a satisfying snack.

12. Popcorn: Air-popped popcorn is a whole grain snack low in calories and high in fiber.

13. Rice Cake with Almond Butter: A rice cake topped with almond butter is a crunchy, satisfying snack with healthy fats and protein.

14. Cherry Tomatoes with Mozzarella: Cherry tomatoes paired with fresh mozzarella cheese provide a combination of vitamins, minerals, and protein.

15. Homemade Energy Balls: Blend dates, nuts, and oats to create homemade energy balls for a quick and nutritious snack.

16. Celery Sticks with Cream Cheese: Celery sticks filled with cream cheese offer a crunchy, low-carb snack option.

17. Sliced Bell Peppers with Guacamole: Sliced bell peppers dipped in guacamole provide fiber, vitamins, and healthy fats.

18. Banana with Almond Butter: A banana smeared with almond butter is a simple and nutritious snack rich in potassium and protein.

19. Seaweed Snacks: Roasted seaweed snacks are low in calories and provide essential minerals like iodine.

20. Frozen Grapes: Frozen grapes make a refreshing and naturally sweet snack that's perfect for hot days.

These snack options offer a balance of nutrients to keep you fueled and satisfied throughout the day. Choose based on your preferences and dietary needs.

Chapter 8

Beverages and Smoothies for Hydration and Nutrition

1. Green Smoothie: Blend spinach, kale, banana, pineapple, and coconut water for a nutritious and hydrating green smoothie.

2. Berry Blast Smoothie: Blend mixed berries (such as strawberries, blueberries, raspberries), Greek yogurt, spinach, and almond milk for a refreshing and antioxidant-rich smoothie.

3. Tropical Fruit Smoothie: Blend mango, pineapple, banana, coconut milk, and a splash of orange juice for a taste of the tropics packed with vitamins and minerals.

4. Watermelon Mint Cooler: Blend fresh watermelon with a few mint leaves and a squeeze of lime for a refreshing and hydrating summer beverage.

5. Cucumber Limeade: Blend cucumber slices with lime juice, honey, and water for a cooling and revitalizing drink.

6. Coconut Water: Enjoy coconut water straight from the coconut or packaged for a natural source of hydration and electrolytes.

7. Iced Green Tea: Brew green tea and chill it in the refrigerator for a refreshing and antioxidant-rich beverage.

8. Chia Seed Lemonade: Mix chia seeds with lemon juice, honey, and water for a hydrating drink with added fiber and nutrients.

9. Ginger Turmeric Tea: Steep fresh ginger and turmeric in hot water for a soothing and anti-inflammatory beverage.

10. Golden Milk: Warm milk (dairy or plant-based) with turmeric, cinnamon, ginger, and a touch of honey for a comforting and nutritious drink.

11. Matcha Latte: Whisk matcha powder with hot water and frothed milk for a vibrant and antioxidant-packed beverage.

12. Berry-Lemon Infused Water: Add sliced berries and lemon to a pitcher of water for a refreshing and hydrating infused water option.

13. Pineapple Coconut Smoothie: Blend pineapple chunks, coconut milk, Greek yogurt, and a handful of spinach for a tropical and creamy smoothie.

14. Kale Apple Smoothie: Blend kale, apple, cucumber, lemon juice, and coconut water for a refreshing and detoxifying green smoothie.

15. Banana Almond Butter Smoothie: Blend banana, almond butter, almond milk, and a dash of cinnamon for a creamy and protein-rich smoothie.

16. Avocado Spinach Smoothie: Blend avocado, spinach, banana, Greek yogurt, and coconut

water for a creamy and nutrient-dense green smoothie.

17. Chocolate Peanut Butter Smoothie: Blend banana, cocoa powder, peanut butter, Greek yogurt, and almond milk for a satisfying and indulgent smoothie.

18. Strawberry Beet Smoothie: Blend strawberries, cooked beetroot, Greek yogurt, and orange juice for a vibrant and nutrient-packed smoothie.

19. Mango Coconut Water Smoothie: Blend mango chunks, coconut water, Greek yogurt, and a squeeze of lime for a refreshing and tropical smoothie.

20. Pomegranate Green Tea: Mix pomegranate juice with chilled green tea for a refreshing and antioxidant-rich beverage.

21. Watermelon Cucumber Cooler: Blend watermelon, cucumber, mint leaves, and lime juice with ice for a hydrating and cooling summer drink.

22. Blueberry Lavender Lemonade: Blend blueberries, lavender, lemon juice, honey, and water for a fragrant and antioxidant-rich lemonade.

23. Peach Ginger Iced Tea: Brew peach tea and add sliced fresh ginger for a refreshing and soothing iced tea option.

24. Raspberry Coconut Water Smoothie: Blend raspberries, coconut water, Greek yogurt, and a splash of vanilla extract for a hydrating and creamy smoothie.

25. Cherry Vanilla Smoothie: Blend cherries, vanilla Greek yogurt, almond milk, and a sprinkle of cinnamon for a delicious and antioxidant-packed smoothie option.

These beverages and smoothies offer a variety of flavors and nutrients to keep you hydrated and nourished throughout the day. Enjoy them as snacks or alongside meals for an extra boost of nutrition.

Chapter 9

Desserts and Treats recipes for Occasional Indulgence

1. Chocolate Avocado Mousse:

Ingredients: Ripe avocados, cocoa powder, honey, vanilla extract.

Method: Blend avocados, cocoa powder, honey, and vanilla extract until smooth. Chill and serve.

2. Banana Nice Cream:

Ingredients: Frozen bananas, almond milk.

Method: Blend frozen bananas with a splash of almond milk until creamy. Serve with toppings.

3. Coconut Macaroons:

Ingredients: Shredded coconut, sweetened condensed milk, vanilla extract.

Method: Mix shredded coconut, sweetened condensed milk, and vanilla extract. Form into balls and bake.

4. Dark Chocolate Truffles:

Ingredients: Dark chocolate, heavy cream, cocoa powder, nuts or coconut for coating.

Method: Mix melted dark chocolate and heavy cream. Let it set, then roll into balls and coat in cocoa powder or chopped nuts.

5. Berry Parfait:

Ingredients: Greek yogurt, mixed berries, granola.

Method: Layer Greek yogurt with mixed berries and granola in a glass.

6. Grilled Fruit Skewers:

Ingredients: Pineapple, peaches, bananas, honey.

Method: Skewer fruit and grill until caramelized. Serve with a drizzle of honey.

7. Chocolate-Dipped Strawberries:

Ingredients: Fresh strawberries, dark chocolate.

Method: Dip strawberries in melted dark chocolate and let them set.

8. Baked Apples with Cinnamon:

Ingredients: Apples, cinnamon, brown sugar, nuts.

Method: Core apples and fill with cinnamon, brown sugar, and nuts. Bake until tender.

9. Mini Cheesecakes:

Ingredients: Cream cheese, sugar, eggs, vanilla extract, fruit compote or chocolate ganache.

Method: Make individual cheesecakes and top with fruit compote or chocolate ganache.

10. Peanut Butter Chocolate Chip Blondies:

Ingredients: Peanut butter, sugar, eggs, vanilla extract, chocolate chips.

Method: Mix ingredients and bake until golden brown.

11. Lemon Bars:

Ingredients: Lemon, sugar, flour, butter, eggs.

Method: Make a lemon filling and pour over a shortbread crust. Bake and dust with powdered sugar.

12. Homemade Ice Cream Sandwiches:

Ingredients: Vanilla ice cream, homemade cookies.

Method: Sandwich ice cream between homemade cookies.

13. Raspberry Sorbet:

Ingredients: Frozen raspberries, lemon juice, honey.

Method: Blend ingredients until smooth. Freeze and serve.

14. Chocolate Covered Pretzels:

Ingredients: Pretzels, dark chocolate.

Method: Dip pretzels in melted chocolate and let them set.

15. Homemade Brownies:

Ingredients: Chocolate, butter, sugar, eggs, flour.

Method: Mix ingredients and bake until set. Cut into squares and serve.

16. Caramel Popcorn:

Ingredients: Popcorn, butter, brown sugar, corn syrup.

Method: Make caramel sauce, pour over popcorn, and bake until coated.

17. Fruit Tart:

Ingredients: Pastry dough, pastry cream, fresh fruit.

Method: Fill baked pastry dough with pastry cream and top with fresh fruit.

18. Chocolate Lava Cake:

Ingredients: Chocolate, butter, sugar, eggs, flour.

Method: Bake until the outside is set but the center is still gooey.

19. Tiramisu:

Ingredients: Ladyfingers, coffee, mascarpone cheese, cocoa powder.

Method: Layer soaked ladyfingers with mascarpone mixture and dust with cocoa powder.

20. Panna Cotta:

Ingredients: Cream, sugar, gelatin, vanilla extract.

Method: Heat cream and sugar, add gelatin and vanilla, pour into molds, and chill until set.

21. Key Lime Pie:

Ingredients: Graham cracker crust, condensed milk, lime juice, eggs.

Method: Mix ingredients and bake until set. Chill and serve with whipped cream.

22. Raspberry Cheesecake Bars:

Ingredients: Cream cheese, sugar, eggs, vanilla extract, raspberry jam.

Method: Make a cheesecake batter, swirl in raspberry jam, and bake until set.

23. Chocolate Mousse Cake:

Ingredients: Chocolate cake, chocolate mousse, whipped cream.

Method: Layer chocolate cake with chocolate mousse and top with whipped cream.

24. Homemade Doughnuts:

Ingredients: Yeast, flour, sugar, milk, butter.

Method: Make dough, let rise, shape into rings, fry, and coat in sugar.

25. Red Velvet Cupcakes:

Ingredients: Red velvet cake mix, cream cheese frosting.

Method: Bake cupcakes, frost with cream cheese frosting, and decorate as desired.

These dessert and treat recipes are perfect for special occasions when you want to indulge in something sweet and satisfying. Enjoy making and sharing these delicious treats!

Chapter 10

Special Dietary Considerations and Modifications

Here are some special dietary considerations and modifications for the desserts and treats mentioned:

1. Gluten-Free Options: Substitute wheat flour with gluten-free flour blends or almond flour in recipes like macaroons, brownies, and fruit tarts. Ensure that other ingredients like baking powder, oats, and flavorings are also gluten-free.

2. Dairy-Free Alternatives: Use dairy-free alternatives such as coconut milk, almond milk, or oat milk in recipes that call for milk or cream. Replace butter with dairy-free margarine or coconut oil. Choose dairy-free

chocolate chips and cream cheese for recipes like cheesecakes and brownies.

3. Vegan Substitutions: Replace eggs with flaxseed or chia seed eggs, mashed bananas, or applesauce in recipes like brownies and muffins. Opt for vegan chocolate chips and cocoa powder in chocolate-based recipes. Use vegan butter or coconut oil instead of regular butter.

4. Reduced Sugar Options: Substitute refined sugar with natural sweeteners like honey, maple syrup, or coconut sugar. Adjust the sweetness to taste and consider using ripe fruits like bananas or dates to sweeten desserts naturally.

5. Nut-Free Alternatives: Replace nuts with seeds like sunflower seeds, pumpkin seeds, or hemp seeds in recipes like granola bars or energy balls. Use seed butter instead of peanut or almond butter for those with nut allergies.

6. Lower-Calorie Variations: Choose lighter ingredients such as Greek yogurt instead of heavy cream in recipes like cheesecakes or mousses. Use less sugar or sugar substitutes like stevia or erythritol to reduce calorie content.

7. Portion Control: Make smaller portion sizes or mini versions of desserts like mini cheesecakes, bite-sized brownies, or mini fruit tarts to help with portion control and moderation.

8. Allergen-Free Options: Be mindful of common allergens like gluten, dairy, nuts, and eggs when preparing desserts for individuals with allergies. Provide alternative options or ensure thorough cleaning of utensils and surfaces to prevent cross-contamination.

9. Customization: Allow for customization by offering a variety of toppings, fillings, or mix-ins so individuals can personalize their desserts according to their dietary preferences and restrictions.

By considering these special dietary considerations and modifications, you can accommodate a variety of dietary needs and preferences while still enjoying delicious desserts and treats. Always double-check ingredient labels and verify with individuals about their specific dietary requirements to ensure everyone can safely enjoy the indulgence.

Chapter 11

Lifestyle Tips for Managing Parkinson's Symptoms Through Nutrition

Managing Parkinson's symptoms through nutrition involves making thoughtful choices to support overall health and well-being. Here are some lifestyle tips:

1. Balanced Diet: Aim for a balanced diet rich in fruits, vegetables, whole grains, lean proteins, and healthy fats. This provides essential nutrients to support overall health and may help manage symptoms.

2. Hydration: Stay hydrated by drinking plenty of water throughout the day. Dehydration can worsen symptoms like constipation and fatigue.

3. Fiber-Rich Foods: Incorporate fiber-rich foods like fruits, vegetables, whole grains, and legumes into your diet to help prevent

constipation, a common symptom of Parkinson's disease.

4. Omega-3 Fatty Acids: Include foods high in omega-3 fatty acids, such as salmon, flaxseeds, chia seeds, and walnuts, which may have anti-inflammatory properties and support brain health.

5. Limit Processed Foods: Minimize consumption of processed foods, sugary snacks, and refined carbohydrates, which can contribute to inflammation and may exacerbate symptoms.

6. Protein Distribution: Distribute protein intake evenly throughout the day to minimize the impact on levodopa absorption. Avoid high-protein meals close to medication times, as they may interfere with medication effectiveness.

7. Antioxidant-Rich Foods: Consume foods rich in antioxidants, such as berries, leafy greens, nuts, and seeds, to help protect against oxidative stress and inflammation.

8. Portion Control: Pay attention to portion sizes to prevent overeating, which can lead to weight gain and worsen symptoms. Use smaller plates and bowls to help control portion sizes.

9. Regular Meals: Eat regular meals and snacks throughout the day to maintain stable blood sugar levels and provide sustained energy.

10. Medication Management: Take medications as prescribed and discuss any concerns or side effects with your healthcare provider. Some medications may interact with certain foods or nutrients.

11. Collaborate with a Dietitian: Consult with a registered dietitian who specializes in Parkinson's disease to develop a personalized nutrition plan tailored to your individual needs and preferences.

12. Mindful Eating: Practice mindful eating by focusing on the sensory experience of eating, chewing food thoroughly, and savoring each

bite. This can enhance digestion and satisfaction with meals.

13. Experiment with Cooking Techniques: Experiment with cooking techniques like steaming, baking, grilling, and sautéing to enhance flavor and texture without adding excessive fat or sodium.

14. Supplement Consideration: Discuss with your healthcare provider whether you need any specific supplements, such as vitamin D or B12, to address potential deficiencies associated with Parkinson's disease or medication use.

15. Social Support: Maintain social connections and enjoy meals with family and friends. Sharing meals can provide emotional support and promote overall well-being.

By incorporating these lifestyle tips into your daily routine, you can optimize nutrition to support your health and manage Parkinson's symptoms more effectively. Always consult with your healthcare provider or a registered dietitian before making significant changes to your diet or lifestyle.

Chapter 12

Resources for Further Reading and Support

Here are some resources for further reading and support on managing Parkinson's disease through nutrition:

1. Parkinson's Foundation: The Parkinson's Foundation offers a variety of resources on nutrition and Parkinson's disease, including articles, webinars, and educational materials. Their website provides valuable information and support for individuals living with Parkinson's and their caregivers. (Website: parkinson.org)

2. Michael J. Fox Foundation: The Michael J. Fox Foundation is a leading organization dedicated to Parkinson's research and support. Their website includes resources on nutrition and Parkinson's, as well as information on clinical trials, advocacy, and community events. (Website: michael j fox.org)

3. National Institute on Aging: The National Institute on Aging (NIA) provides resources on healthy aging, including information on nutrition for older adults and those with chronic conditions like Parkinson's disease. Their website offers tips, articles, and research updates related to nutrition and aging. (Website: nia.nih.gov)

4. American Parkinson Disease Association (APDA): The APDA offers educational resources, support groups, and wellness programs for individuals affected by Parkinson's disease. Their website includes information on nutrition, exercise, and managing symptoms, as well as links to local resources and events. (Website: apdaparkinson.org)

5. Academy of Nutrition and Dietetics: The Academy of Nutrition and Dietetics is a professional organization for registered dietitians and nutrition professionals. Their website provides evidence-based information on nutrition for various health conditions,

including Parkinson's disease. You can find articles, fact sheets, and tips for optimizing nutrition and managing symptoms. (Website: eatright.org)

6. Books: There are several books available on Parkinson's disease and nutrition written by healthcare professionals and experts in the field. Some recommended titles include "Parkinson's Disease and Movement Disorders: Nutritional Therapies" by Lieberman and Shukla, and "Eat Well, Stay Well with Parkinson's Disease" by Kathrynne Holden.

7. Support Groups: Joining a local or online support group for individuals living with Parkinson's disease can provide valuable peer support, practical tips, and shared experiences related to nutrition and lifestyle management. Websites like Parkinson.org and MichaelJFox.org offer directories of support groups.

8. Consult a Registered Dietitian: Consider consulting with a registered dietitian who

specializes in Parkinson's disease or neurological conditions. A dietitian can provide personalized nutrition counseling, meal planning guidance, and support to help you optimize your diet and manage symptoms effectively.

These resources offer valuable information, support, and guidance for individuals living with Parkinson's disease and their caregivers. It's important to stay informed and empowered in managing your health and well-being.

Chapter 13

Frequently Asked Questions

Here are some frequently asked questions about Parkinson's disease:

1. What is Parkinson's disease?

Parkinson's disease is a progressive neurodegenerative disorder that affects movement. It occurs when nerve cells in the brain that produce dopamine become impaired or die, leading to symptoms such as tremors, stiffness, slowness of movement, and balance problems.

2. What causes Parkinson's disease?

The exact cause of Parkinson's disease is unknown, but it is believed to involve a combination of genetic and environmental factors. Some research suggests that exposure to certain toxins or chemicals may increase the risk of developing Parkinson's disease.

3. What are the symptoms of Parkinson's disease?

Common symptoms of Parkinson's disease include tremors, bradykinesia (slowness of movement), rigidity (stiffness), postural instability (balance problems), and changes in speech and writing. Other symptoms may include loss of smell, sleep disturbances, depression, and cognitive changes.

4. Is there a cure for Parkinson's disease?
Currently, there is no cure for Parkinson's disease. Treatment focuses on managing symptoms and improving quality of life. Medications, physical therapy, speech therapy, and lifestyle modifications are commonly used to manage symptoms.

5. How is Parkinson's disease diagnosed?
Parkinson's disease is diagnosed based on medical history, physical examination, and assessment of symptoms. There is no definitive test for Parkinson's disease, so diagnosis is often made based on the presence of characteristic symptoms and ruling out other conditions that may cause similar symptoms.

6. What is the role of medication in treating Parkinson's disease?
Medications used to treat Parkinson's disease aim to increase dopamine levels in the brain, reduce symptoms, and improve motor function. Common medications include levodopa, dopamine agonists, MAO-B inhibitors, and COMT inhibitors.

Medication regimens are tailored to individual symptoms and may need adjustment over time.

7. Are there lifestyle changes that can help manage Parkinson's disease?

Yes, lifestyle changes such as regular exercise, physical therapy, speech therapy, and nutritional support can help manage symptoms and improve quality of life for individuals with Parkinson's disease. Maintaining a healthy diet, staying hydrated, getting enough sleep, and managing stress are also important.

8. What is deep brain stimulation (DBS), and how is it used to treat Parkinson's disease?

Deep brain stimulation (DBS) is a surgical procedure that involves implanting electrodes into specific areas of the brain to help regulate abnormal brain activity associated with Parkinson's disease. DBS can help improve motor symptoms and reduce the need for medication in some individuals with Parkinson's disease.

9. What is the prognosis for Parkinson's disease?

Parkinson's disease is a progressive disorder, meaning symptoms typically worsen over time. However, the progression of the disease varies from person to person, and not everyone will experience the same symptoms or rate of progression. With proper treatment and management, many individuals with Parkinson's disease can lead fulfilling lives for many years after diagnosis.

10. Where can I find support and resources for Parkinson's disease?

Organizations such as the Parkinson's Foundation, the Michael J. Fox Foundation, and local support groups provide resources, educational materials, and support services for individuals living with Parkinson's disease and their caregivers. Additionally, healthcare providers, including neurologists and movement disorder specialists, can offer guidance and support tailored to individual needs.

These are just a few of the frequently asked questions about Parkinson's disease. If you or someone you know is affected by Parkinson's disease, it's important to seek guidance from healthcare professionals and trusted organizations for personalized information and support.